OSTEOPOROSIS PREVENTION DIET

Purposeful Diet For Stronger Bone Health. Recipes Cookbook On Knowledge To Live Well, Manage, Strive And Reverse Bone Weakness

DR. CHARLSE BLESSING

DISCLAIMER

The information in this book is meant solely for educational reasons. This book's contents are not meant to be used in place of expert medical advice, diagnosis, or treatment. Any decisions you make about your health must be discussed with a licensed healthcare provider.

Every effort has been made by the author to guarantee that the material in this book is correct and current as of the date of publication. Still, since medical knowledge advances rapidly, new studies might be conducted that change our understanding this illness and how best to manage it with food.

This book may contains references to and mentions of various people, things, websites, organizations, and other entities that the author does not support, advocate, or have any association with.

There is no implied sponsorship or collaboration; all references and remarks are made only for informational purposes.

In order to address their individual health concerns, readers are advised to independently verify any information contained in this book and to consult with healthcare specialists. Any negative effects arising from the use or implementation of the material in this book, whether direct or indirect, are not the responsibility of the author or the publisher.

The dietary suggestions and counsel provided in this book are broad in scope and might not be appropriate for every individual. Readers are recommended to seek tailored counsel from trained healthcare specialists as individual health problems and demands differ.

The reader accepts the conditions of this disclaimer by reading this book.

FACTS ABOUT THIS BOOK

The "Osteoporosis Prevention Diet" book is a comprehensive resource for anyone wishing to enhance bone health and reduce their risk of osteoporosis through dietary practices. The introduction covers the goals of the book, provides a broad overview of osteoporosis, and emphasizes the vital role that diet plays in prevention. The second section lays the foundation for a more knowledgeable approach to prevention by going over the basics of osteoporosis, its causes, and its broader effects on overall health.

The book primarily examines the nutrients required for bone health, emphasizing the significance of calcium, vitamin D, and other critical elements. The article then guides how to design a personalized diet plan that will prevent osteoporosis by including foods high in calcium, arranging nutrients on a plate in a way that ensures an adequate intake of vitamin D, and cooking meals.

A thorough analysis of foods that are vital for healthy bone development is presented, using a broad perspective. These foods include both plant-based substitutes and conventional dairy sources. As the role of hydration in preserving bone density is examined, the importance of water and specific beverages in improving overall well-being is emphasized.

The book discusses the vital role exercise plays in preventing osteoporosis and covers weight-bearing and resistance exercises, flexibility training, and balance training. A thorough examination of lifestyle factors that affect bone health is included, such as drinking alcohol, smoking, managing stress, and getting adequate sleep. This preventive strategy has several facets.

Advice is offered on the necessity of supplements and how to take them responsibly, with a focus on the importance of consulting medical professionals. Because it includes recipes specifically created for healthy bones and takes into consideration different life seasons, the book is both flexible and beneficial.

In addition to offering short-term dietary suggestions, the book also looks at how sustainable these changes might be and offers guidance on developing long-term routines. The last section summarizes the key takeaways, expresses optimism for a better future, and stresses the need for goal-setting, motivating others, and carrying on with preventative actions for bone health. When everything is said and done, the "Osteoporosis Prevention Diet" is an invaluable resource that provides people with the information and practical strategies they need to maintain long-term bone health.

CHAPTER ONE

INTRODUCTION
A Synopsis of Bone Loss

Osteoporosis is a common and potentially debilitating medical disorder characterized by bone weakening that raises the risk of fractures. This disease, which affects both sexes equally, is particularly prevalent in older people. As bone mass and density decrease, bones become weaker and more porous. Osteoporosis is usually associated with senior age, although it can also affect younger people for several causes, such as hormone imbalances, poor diet, and sedentary lifestyles.

The main consequence of osteoporosis is a heightened risk of fractures, especially in weight-bearing bones like the hips, spine, and wrists. These fractures can cause discomfort, limited mobility, and even greater death rates, which can have a huge detrimental impact on an individual's quality of life, particularly for elderly people. Understanding the origins, risk factors, and preventive measures of osteoporosis is crucial for managing and reducing its effects.

The Benefits of Nutritional Guidance

Diet has a major role in managing and preventing osteoporosis. A healthy diet ensures that the body receives the minerals it needs, including calcium and vitamin D, which are essential for strong bones. Maintaining bone production requires calcium, and vitamin D facilitates the absorption of calcium by the intestines. A well-balanced diet that includes enough levels of these components as well as other vitamins and minerals is advised to maintain optimal bone density and strength.

Apart from calcium and vitamin D, magnesium, phosphorus, and vitamin K are also necessary nutrients for strong bones. Moreover, a diet rich in fruits, vegetables, and whole grains contains antioxidants and phytochemicals that support bone health as well as overall wellness. In addition to focusing on specific nutrients, dietary prevention of osteoporosis is a complete approach that considers the synergistic effects of several food components.

The Purpose of the Osteoporosis Prevention Diet Book

The Osteoporosis Prevention Diet Book aims to arm readers with the knowledge and tools necessary to take control of their bone health through wise food choices. The book's objective is to educate readers on the specific nutrients needed for healthy bones and how to incorporate them into their daily diets. It provides practical guidance on meal planning that enables people to meet nutritional needs without compromising taste or variety.

Furthermore, the book clears up misconceptions and provides factual information on widely held notions about nutrition and osteoporosis. It emphasizes how important healthy lifestyle choices—consistent exercise and maintaining a healthy weight—combine with a diet that promotes strong bones. By encouraging a proactive and informed approach to osteoporosis prevention, the ultimate goal is to enable people to take charge of their bone health and reduce their risk of fractures as they age.

CHAPTER TWO

UNDERSTANDING OSTEOPOROSIS
Foundations of Bone Health

Bone health is essential to general health because bones store essential nutrients, support important organs, and offer structural support. A person's skeleton undergoes constant alterations during their lifespan due to the breakdown and regeneration of their bones. An abundance of minerals, such as calcium and phosphorus, in the diet, are necessary to maintain bone strength and density. Regular exercise, especially weight-bearing exercises, promotes bone formation and is beneficial to bone health.

The intricate arrangement of minerals and collagen that constitutes bones endows them with robustness and durability. Understanding the need for a well-balanced diet with enough quantities of calcium and vitamin D is necessary to maintain good bone health. Vitamin D, which aids in the body's absorption of calcium, and calcium are the building blocks of bone. Together, they form a strong team that protects against illnesses like osteoporosis and preserves bone density.

Causes and Risk Factors of Osteoporosis

Bones that are weak and porous are the hallmarks of osteoporosis, a disease of the bone-rebuilding process. The development of osteoporosis is caused by several factors. Aging is a significant risk factor due to age-related decreases in bone density. Because hormones diminish estrogen levels, especially in postmenopausal women, they may accelerate bone loss.

Nutritional deficiencies can affect the health of your bones, particularly those related to calcium and vitamin D. Many medications, such as glucocorticoids and some anticonvulsants, may be connected to bone loss. Lifestyle variables that raise the risk of osteoporosis include excessive alcohol consumption, smoking, and sedentary behavior.

An individual's susceptibility to osteoporosis is influenced by their genetic composition. A larger chance of contracting the sickness oneself may exist for those with a family history of it. Ethnicity has an impact on risk as well; Caucasians and Asians are more susceptible.

The Impact of Osteoporosis on Overall Health

Osteoporosis affects not just the skeletal system but also general health. More severe bone fractures can cause significant morbidity and death. Higher mortality rates are associated with fractures, particularly those of the hip because of complications such as blood clots and pneumonia.

Because osteoporosis reduces bone density, a person may become shorter and adopt a stooped posture. These physical changes can hurt a person's looks, mobility, and independence. A person's mental and overall well-being may be adversely impacted by osteoporosis, which frequently causes persistent discomfort and a lower quality of life.

Furthermore, fractures related to osteoporosis can significantly increase healthcare costs since patients may require extended hospital admissions, rehabilitation, and ongoing medical care. Reducing the consequences of osteoporosis on bones and overall health requires preventive measures. These consist of frequent weight-bearing exercise, a well-balanced diet rich in calcium and vitamin D, and lifestyle modifications.

CHAPTER THREE

SUPPLEMENTS IN DIET REQUIRED FOR STRONG BONES

Calcium: The Building Block of Strong Bones

Since calcium is necessary to maintain the density and structural integrity of bones, it is without a doubt the foundation of bone health. This mineral is an important part of bone tissue and regulates several physiological processes, including blood coagulation, muscle contraction, and nerve transmission. Making sure you are getting adequate calcium in your diet is essential for preventing osteoporosis.

However, calcium must come from diet because the human body is unable to produce it on its own. Dairy items like milk, yogurt, and cheese are rich in calcium. If you can't digest dairy or don't want to eat it, fortified plant milk, leafy greens like broccoli and kale, and some fish like salmon and sardines can be excellent alternatives.

Maintaining a healthy calcium intake is crucial since excessive calcium consumption can lead to kidney stones and other issues. It's also critical to keep in mind that several factors, including age, gender, and hormonal changes, might impact the absorption of calcium. Vitamin D, which is also necessary for strong bones, should be taken with foods high in calcium for optimal effects.

Vitamin D: Aiding in the Body's Calcium Absorption

In particular, vitamin D has a critical role in promoting the absorption and utilization of calcium, making it a necessary component of any osteoporosis prevention diet. What makes this fat-soluble vitamin unique is that it can be produced by the body in reaction to sun exposure. A few factors can interfere with the body's natural production of vitamin D, such as the use of sunscreen, aging-related changes in skin metabolism, and insufficient sun exposure.

Dietary sources of vitamin D include egg yolks, fortified foods like various cereals and dairy products, and fatty fish (like salmon and mackerel). For those who don't get enough sun exposure or have problems getting enough vitamin D from their diet, supplements could be suggested. Because vitamin D enhances calcium absorption in the small intestine and aids in blood calcium regulation, calcium and vitamin D complement each other well.

Extra Vital Nutrients for Strong Bones

Many other minerals, in addition to calcium and vitamin D, are essential for preserving the health and density of bones. For instance, magnesium supports healthy bone growth and development and helps convert vitamin D into its active form. Good sources of magnesium include whole grains, nuts, and seeds, as well as leafy green vegetables.

Phosphorus is a crucial mineral that strengthens teeth and bones and works in concert with calcium to maintain bone structure. There is a lot of phosphorus in meat, dairy, and nuts. Sufficient consumption of this mineral is necessary for healthy, strong bones in general.

Furthermore, vitamin K is necessary for the creation of proteins that regulate bone metabolism and mineralization. Leafy green vegetables, such as kale and spinach, are great sources of vitamin K.

In conclusion, a well-rounded diet that goes beyond just calcium and vitamin D can help prevent osteoporosis by incorporating a variety of nutrients that all work together to support good bone health. A well-balanced diet high in these vital nutrients can help people maintain a stronger skeleton and reduce their risk of osteoporosis and related fractures.

CHAPTER FOUR

FORMULATING A NUTRITION PROGRAM TO PREVENT OSTEOPOROSIS

Building a Balanced and Nutrient-Rich Plate:

A well-balanced plate full of nutrients is the first step in developing a diet that prevents osteoporosis. Giving the body the nutrition it needs to sustain healthy bones requires a balanced meal. Ensure that your plate includes a variety of food groups, such as whole grains, fruits, vegetables, lean meats, and healthy fats.

These components work together to offer a broad spectrum of vitamins and minerals that are critical for maintaining bone density.

The vitamins and antioxidants present in fruits and vegetables support overall health and bone health. A rainbow of veggies ensures a broad range of vitamins and minerals that promote healthy bones. Whole grains provide fiber, complex carbohydrates, and important minerals including magnesium, which is necessary for bone metabolism. Lean proteins, which are present in fish, poultry, tofu, and lentils, provide essential amino acids that are necessary for the upkeep and regeneration of bone tissue.

In addition to macronutrients, healthy fats—such as those found in nuts, avocados, and olive oil—are necessary for the absorption of fat-soluble vitamins, such as vitamin D, which is important for bone health. Putting together a plate with a variety of nutrient-dense meals is the first step toward a diet that helps prevent osteoporosis.

Including Calcium-Rich Foods:

Calcium is essential for maintaining healthy bones since it is a fundamental building block of new bone. Maintaining bone mass and reducing the risk of fractures require consuming an adequate amount of calcium from your diet. Non-dairy forms of calcium can also be beneficial for those who follow a plant-based diet or are lactose intolerant, even though dairy products like milk, yogurt, and cheese are well-known sources of the mineral.

Leafy green vegetables such as broccoli, bok choy, and others are excellent sources of calcium. Consuming foods like cereals and plant-based milk replacements that have been fortified can also help you improve your consumption of calcium. You may meet your daily calcium requirements by including a variety of these foods in your meals.

Balance is just as important for strong bones as calcium. If one takes excessive amounts of calcium supplements without considering other dietary factors, such as vitamin D levels, the outcome can not be what is intended or even dangerous. As a result, it is suggested to employ a thorough strategy that incorporates a variety of foods strong in calcium.

Making Enough Vitamin D-Rich Meals:

Since vitamin D is essential for the absorption of calcium, it is a critical component of a diet that prevents osteoporosis. Although vitamin D is produced by the body naturally when exposed to sunshine, dietary sources are equally crucial, especially for those with restricted diets or little sun exposure.

Fish high in omega-3 fatty acids, such as salmon and mackerel, are excellent sources of vitamin D. Orange juice, certain dairy products, and breakfast cereals are a few fortified foods that may help you consume more vitamin D. By improving the absorption of calcium, you can support bone health by incorporating these foods into your meals.

However, as consuming too much vitamin D can be dangerous, it's imperative to strike a balance. As a result, it's important to carefully control the combination of dietary sources, sun exposure, and, if needed, supplementation to maintain adequate vitamin D levels.

In summary, creating a well-balanced plate, including foods high in calcium, and cooking meals with adequate amounts of vitamin D are all crucial components of a diet that successfully avoids osteoporosis. By following specific dietary recommendations, people can take proactive steps to maintain strong and healthy bones throughout their lifetimes.

CHAPTER FIVE

FOODS TO EAT FOR OPTIMAL BONE HEALTH
Dairy and Non-Dairy Sources of Calcium:

A varied diet rich in foods high in calcium is essential for preventing osteoporosis. To maintain the best possible bone health, this mineral is essential. One prominent feature of traditional dairy products is that they are the primary source of calcium. These consist of cheese, yogurt, and milk. They provide this mineral in an extremely absorbable form that strengthens and densely coats bones. It's crucial to keep in mind that some people may not be able to tolerate lactose or may choose non-dairy alternatives for a variety of reasons, such as nutritional or ethical concerns.

For those attempting to prevent osteoporosis, a well-balanced diet that includes calcium from non-dairy sources is vital. When seeking for a plant-based alternative, broccoli and other leafy greens provide a high calcium content. Plant-based milks that have been fortified, such as rice, soy, or almond milk, can be good sources of calcium. Not only are these alternatives good for those following a restricted diet, but they also provide a range of flavors and textures that make utilizing them in different recipes easier.

It is important to consider these dietary sources in addition to the overall nutritional balance in the diet. A sufficient intake of vitamin D is necessary for the absorption of calcium and the preservation of bone health. To ensure they get the daily necessary dosage of calcium for strong, healthy bones, people should focus on eating a balanced diet that includes a variety of dairy and non-dairy calcium sources.

Sunlight exposure is a crucial component of a diet meant to prevent osteoporosis, yet it's often overlooked. The sun's ultraviolet B (UVB) rays, or sunshine, cause the skin to generate vitamin D. This vitamin is necessary for calcium absorption and strong bones. To maintain optimal levels of vitamin D, it is essential to incorporate sunlight exposure into one's daily routine, particularly in the morning when UVB rays are most abundant.

Even yet, some people won't be able to survive just on sunshine, especially in the winter or in places with limited sunlight. Therefore, including dietary sources of vitamin D in the osteoporosis preventative diet is essential. Good sources of vitamin D include egg yolks, fortified dairy, and plant-based milk, and fatty fish such as mackerel and salmon. Furthermore, for those who struggle to obtain adequate amounts of nutrients from diet and sunshine, vitamin D supplements may be recommended.

Maintaining a balance between sun exposure and dietary sources of vitamin D is crucial for an overall osteoporosis preventive plan. Ensuring that individuals obtain adequate vitamin D from both sunlight and food supplements, reduces the risk of deficiency and enhances overall bone health.

Plant-Based Alternatives for Bone Nutrition:

Plant-based options for bone feeding have drawn a lot of attention as more and more people choose vegetarian or vegan diets. Even though conventional sources of calcium and vitamin D are usually associated with animal products, it's crucial to investigate plant-based alternatives to meet the dietary needs of those who are worried about preventing osteoporosis within their dietary preferences.

Plants that contain leafy green vegetables are an excellent source of calcium. Kale, collard greens, and bok choy are a few examples of them. These foods provide a substantial amount of calcium together with other essential nutrients including vitamin K, which is involved in bone metabolism. Fortified plant-based milk, tofu, and fortified cereals provide additional sources of calcium and vitamin D for plant-based diet followers.

To further enhance bone nourishment, plant-based diets need to include foods strong in magnesium. Nuts, seeds, whole grains, and legumes are good sources of magnesium. Magnesium helps the body absorb calcium, which supports healthy bones. A well-planned plant-based diet that includes a variety of these foods can help people maintain optimal bone health while adhering to their dietary choices.

~ 37 ~

CHAPTER SIX

WATER AND THE CONDITION OF YOUR BONES
Water Is Necessary to Maintain Bone Density:

Water is a vital component of the body that maintains all bodily functions, including bone health. Although it's commonly overlooked in discussions about bone density, staying hydrated is crucial for preserving and improving bone health. Approximately 25% of bones are composed of water, so maintaining adequate hydration is crucial for the proper function of the cells that rebuild bones.

Dehydration may have a detrimental effect on bone density. The body may prioritize supplying water to essential organs when it is dehydrated, which may have an impact on the functionality of bone cells. In addition to causing an imbalance in electrolytes, dehydration can also affect the absorption of minerals like magnesium and calcium, which are crucial for healthy bones. A vital first step for anyone attempting to prevent osteoporosis is maintaining an appropriate hydration intake.

Ensuring we are getting enough water becomes increasingly more crucial as we age. Age-related decreases in the body's water content may increase the risk of bone-related issues. Therefore, adopting a proactive hydration approach is essential for preserving bone density and preventing illnesses like osteoporosis.

Drinks to Support Healthy Bones:

Certain beverages have a special impact on bone health and can help prevent osteoporosis, even if water is still necessary for staying hydrated and maintaining overall health. Because milk contains significant levels of calcium and vitamin D, two elements essential to the mineralization and strength of bones, it is a well-known diet that promotes healthy bones. Other dairy products like cheese and yogurt also include these vital minerals.

Fortified plant-based milk alternatives, such as almond or soy milk, can be excellent sources of calcium and vitamin D in addition to dairy for people who are lactose intolerant or follow a vegan diet. Bone health benefits have also been associated with green tea. It contains polyphenols, which may help to both stop bone resorption and encourage bone development.

It's critical to take drinks' whole nutritional content into account. Drinks with a lot of sugar and caffeine may be bad for your bones. Overindulgence in caffeine can result in calcium excretion in the urine, which could have an impact on bone density. Therefore, individuals who wish to preserve optimal bone health should pay particular attention to beverages that provide essential nutrients without compromising overall nutritional balance.

Sustaining Adequate Hydration for General Well-being:

Sustaining enough hydration goes beyond just drinking enough water; it involves considering a person's overall health, including their diet, degree of physical activity, and lifestyle choices. It is crucial to maintain a balanced diet full of nutrients that support bone health and plenty of water to prevent osteoporosis.

Physical activity has a major impact on bone health, and exercise and hydration are closely associated. Exercise causes sweating, so it's important to drink enough water to stay hydrated. Consuming foods high in water content, such as fruits and vegetables, can also aid in maintaining general hydration. Together with water, these meals provide essential vitamins and minerals that support bone health.

To maintain appropriate hydration levels, it's also imperative to limit dehydrating substances like alcohol and caffeine. The body's ability to retain water can be impacted by alcohol, and an excessive caffeine intake can increase urine production and lead to dehydration.

CHAPTER SEVEN

THE ROLE OF EXERCISE IN OSTEOPOROSIS PREVENTION
Weight-Bearing and Resistance Exercises:

Resistance training and weightlifting are vital components of osteoporosis prevention exercises. These exercises are crucial for maintaining bone density and promoting bone formation in those who are at risk of osteoporosis. Running, trekking, and other activities requiring your bones and muscles to defy gravity are examples of weight-bearing exercises. Over time, the stress from these activities leads the bones to reorganize and become denser. Resistance workouts, on the other hand, use weights or resistance bands to build muscles and bones.

Because resistance training builds bone density and muscle strength, it is particularly beneficial. This is critical because stronger muscles better support the bones, reducing the risk of fractures and falls. Weight-bearing and resistance exercises should be tailored to an individual's fitness level and increased progressively over time to ensure safety and effectiveness. Including these exercises regularly in your routine will significantly aid in the prevention of osteoporosis.

Exercises for Flexibility and Balance Included:

Exercise for flexibility and balance is crucial to an osteoporosis-prevention diet. As adults age, maintaining flexibility and balance is essential to avoiding fractures and falls. Two examples of flexibility exercises that promote preserving a full range of motion in the joints, improving agility, and reducing the risk of injury are yoga and stretching. Yoga in particular is beneficial since it improves flexibility and aids with relaxation and balance.

The main focus of balance training is on exercises that increase coordination and stability since they reduce the chance of falls. Simple exercises like heel-to-toe walks, one-leg stands, and uneven surface balancing drills can significantly improve balance. By including these exercises in a comprehensive program for preventing osteoporosis, individuals can enhance their motor function and reduce their risk of fracture-related occurrences.

Creating a Comprehensive Fitness Program:

A comprehensive fitness program is essential for maintaining overall health and preventing osteoporosis. This routine should include weight-bearing workouts, resistance training, flexibility exercises, and balance training. When combined, these components strengthen bones and reduce the likelihood of osteoporosis-related issues. They also address different aspects of physical well-being.

Variability is crucial in a comprehensive exercise regimen. It is made sure that every aspect of physical health is taken care of by mixing aerobic workouts with weight training and exercises that improve balance and flexibility. In addition to assisting in the prevention of osteoporosis, this technique enhances mental health, cardiovascular health, and weight management.

CHAPTER EIGHT

FACTORS IN LIFESTYLE THAT AFFECT BONE HEALTH
Smoking and Alcohol Use: Impacts on Bone Density

Lifestyle decisions that negatively affect bone health and increase the risk of osteoporosis include smoking and binge drinking. For instance, there is evidence linking smoking to a reduction in bone density. The harmful compounds in cigarette smoke, such as cadmium and nicotine, disturb the delicate balance between bone formation and resorption.

For instance, the cell responsible for bone growth, the osteoblast, is suppressed by nicotine, which lowers bone mass. By obstructing the absorption of calcium, a mineral required for strong bones, smoking also compromises bone health.

Bone density can also be negatively impacted by binge drinking. Prolonged heavy drinking may impair the body's ability to absorb calcium and vitamin D, two essential nutrients for maintaining bone health. A decrease in bone mass may also result from alcohol's disruption of the hormonal balance that regulates the growth of new bones.

Furthermore, drinking too much alcohol might increase the risk of falls and fractures, particularly in the elderly. People who wish to prevent osteoporosis must make better choices and be mindful of their alcohol and tobacco use to preserve their bone health.

Controlling Stress to Promote Better Bone Health

Chronic stress is one of the risk factors for osteoporosis, emphasizing the intricate connection between the body and mind. Extended periods of stress trigger the body to release cortisol, a hormone that can lead to excessive bone loss.

By promoting osteoclast activity, or the disintegration of bone tissue, and inhibiting osteoblast activity, elevated cortisol levels interfere with the process of making new bone. Additionally, stress can exacerbate unhealthy lifestyle choices, such as eating badly and not exercising, which can deteriorate bone health even more.

Thus, efficient stress management is a crucial component of an osteoporosis prevention plan. Lowering cortisol levels and improving wellbeing can be achieved by practicing relaxation techniques including yoga, deep breathing exercises, and meditation.

Regular physical activity also has the added benefit of strengthening bones and reducing stress. By adopting holistic stress management techniques, people can reduce their risk of developing osteoporosis and contribute to maintaining optimal bone health.

Sleeping Enough to Promote the Best Bone Regeneration

Maintaining excellent bone health requires getting adequate sleep, which is an important but sometimes overlooked factor. While we sleep, the body repairs and renews itself, and this also applies to the bones.

Getting adequate sleep is necessary for the release of growth hormone, which is necessary for bone remodeling and growth. Sleep cycle disruptions, such as insomnia or inconsistent sleep patterns, can lead to a decrease in growth hormone secretion, which can hurt bone density.

Moreover, a decrease in sleep has been associated with an increase in cortisol levels, the stress hormone previously discussed. Elevations in cortisol not only lead to bone loss but also disrupt the equilibrium of other hormones vital to strong bones.

Creating a comfortable sleep environment, managing sleep disturbances, and establishing consistent sleep habits are all essential for ensuring optimal bone regeneration. By prioritizing good sleep hygiene, individuals can support the body's natural bone-building processes and contribute to a comprehensive osteoporosis prevention plan.

CHAPTER NINE

VITAMINS AND OSTEOPOROSIS PREVENTION
Acknowledging the Need for Supplements

Osteoporosis prevention involves a multifaceted strategy to maintain bone health, and understanding the role of supplements is crucial. Two of the most crucial elements in this quest are calcium and vitamin D. Calcium is the primary mineral that provides bones their strength and structure, while vitamin D facilitates the body's absorption of calcium. Getting enough of these nutrients through diet alone can often be challenging, especially for those with specific dietary requirements or limited sun exposure (which is a natural source of vitamin D).

By making up for any dietary gaps in essential nutrients, supplements guarantee that the body receives enough of these key elements for healthy bones. Calcium supplements come in a variety of forms, such as calcium carbonate and citrate, and each has special qualities for absorption. Supplemental vitamin D is often recommended, particularly for individuals with conditions that limit their ability to absorb enough amounts of the vitamin or for those who may have difficulty getting enough sunlight.

To maintain strong bones, several micronutrients are necessary in addition to calcium and vitamin D. Trace elements including zinc and copper, magnesium, and vitamin K affect bone density and overall skeletal integrity. An osteoporosis-preventative diet, when paired with other nutrients, can help people age with conserved bone mass and a decreased risk of fractures.

Choosing and Using Supplements Wisely

Choosing and utilizing supplements should be done with caution, even though they may be beneficial. Because not all supplements are created equal, it's critical to consider dosage, quality, and bioavailability. For example, taking calcium supplements with meals promotes optimal absorption. Calcium carbonate or citrate may be preferred depending on considerations such as stomach acidity.

Vitamin D supplements, on the other hand, need to be taken in the prescribed dosage and manner. The active form of vitamin D3, cholecalciferol, has varying suggested dosages based on individual needs and medical conditions. Compared to vitamin D2 (ergocalciferol), it is more efficient. It is always advisable to speak with a healthcare professional to determine the best supplement regimen for your specific requirements.

It is important to thoroughly consider any possible interactions between medications and supplements. As some medications may interfere with the absorption or use of certain nutrients, it is crucial to seek professional assistance to avoid adverse effects. Moreover, obtaining nutrients from whole foods is still an essential part of a balanced approach to osteoporosis prevention; supplements should be used in addition to, not in place of, a nutrient-rich diet.

Talking with Specialists in Medicine

To prevent osteoporosis, it is essential to consult with medical professionals before beginning a supplement regimen. It is necessary to perform thorough assessments of each person's needs, health, and potential drug interactions. Healthcare providers can conduct tests to determine baseline nutritional levels and then tailor suggestions to each patient's specific needs.

Regular monitoring is essential to ensure that selected supplements complement overall health objectives and to make required dosage adjustments. Healthcare professionals can guide how long to take supplements, potential side effects, and the significance of lifestyle changes such as exercise when using supplements.

In summary, a comprehensive approach to osteoporosis prevention includes being aware of the necessity of supplements, carefully choosing and utilizing them, and consulting with medical professionals. This proactive approach empowers individuals to take charge of their bone health by identifying and correcting any deficiencies and optimizing nutritional support for strong and resilient bones.

CHAPTER TEN

RECIPES TO STRENGTHEN YOUR BONES
Breakfasts that Encourage Strong Bones

Breakfasts that promote strong bones are a crucial component of a diet meant to ward off osteoporosis. It is essential to include meals high in essential minerals, like calcium and vitamin D, as these are necessary for the growth and maintenance of bones. A bowl of cereal enriched with milk, which provides calcium and vitamin D, is a classic example. Yogurt with fruits and nuts is another fantastic alternative. These nutrients, which include calcium, protein, and phosphorus, are necessary for strong bones. Oatmeal and other whole grains can enhance the nutritional profile because they contain minerals like magnesium and zinc that support bone density.

Eggs are also a wonderful source of vitamin D and protein. It can be delicious and beneficial to your bones to include eggs in your breakfast meals. In addition to adding taste to a vegetarian omelet, spinach and mushrooms also supply additional minerals including potassium and vitamin K. These breakfast options give you the fundamental components of bone strength, which helps prevent osteoporosis by promoting a balanced diet.

Nutrient-Dense Lunch and Dinner Options

Dietary planning for the prevention of osteoporosis should include nutrient-dense lunch and dinner alternatives in addition to breakfast. Leafy greens are rich in calcium and vitamin K, which are necessary for the mineralization of bones. Examples of these are kale and collard greens. Grilled salmon or other fatty seafood is a fantastic source of vitamin D and omega-3 fatty acids, which help bone density and general skeletal health. One of the best ways to get protein and essential minerals like magnesium and phosphorus is to include beans and legumes in your meals.

For lunch, a quinoa salad with a variety of colorful vegetables and a dollop of feta cheese can supply several minerals that help to build stronger bones. Dinner might be baked sweet potatoes, which are an excellent source of vitamin A and encourage the formation of bone cells. They go well with lean proteins, like grilled chicken or tofu, to make a well-balanced meal that supports strong bones.

Snacks and Desserts to Increase Bone Density

It's not necessary to give up snacks and sweets to keep strong bones. A well-considered choice can satisfy a savory or sweet tooth while boosting bone density. Almonds and other nuts are not only a convenient snack food, but they are also a wonderful source of magnesium, calcium, and vitamin E. A trail mix containing dried fruits and seeds can be a nutritious and palatable midday snack that promotes bone health because it contains a variety of essential elements.

Desserts made with dairy or fortified plant-based milk can be wise choices. A yogurt parfait with layers of fruit and granola can be a tasty treat that promotes bone health because of its calcium and vitamin D content. In addition to gratifying sweet cravings, combining dark chocolate with almonds provides magnesium and other nutrients necessary for strong bones.

In summary, selecting meals for breakfasts, lunches, dinners, snacks, and desserts that highlight the components that are most crucial for strong bones is part of a well-rounded diet that avoids osteoporosis. By adopting a wide variety of meals, people can create a delicious and effective plan to strengthen their bones and reduce their risk of osteoporosis.

CHAPTER ELEVEN

CONSUMPTION ABOUT STAGE OF LIFE
Diets Of Children And Teenagers To Avoid Osteoporosis:

To prevent osteoporosis in the future, it is essential to maintain optimal bone health throughout childhood and adolescence. Because calcium and vitamin D are essential for the development of bones, young people's diets should include dairy products, leafy green vegetables, and fortified meals. Getting enough exercise is just as important because weight-bearing exercises promote bone density. In addition to strengthening their bones, sports, running, and jumping help kids form lifetime habits for a healthy lifestyle.

Reducing the quantity of sugar-filled and carbonated beverages you drink is also essential, since an excess of these may impair your body's capacity to absorb calcium and deplete your stocks of bone mineral. Teaching parents and other caregivers the value of a balanced diet and regular bone health checkups for their children lays the groundwork for lifetime bone strength.

Strategies for Bone Health in Adults and Seniors:

As people mature and reach later phases of life, maintaining bone health becomes increasingly important to prevent osteoporosis. A diet rich in calcium, vitamin D, and other essential minerals is still important, but there may be times when adjustments are needed due to changing absorption capacities and nutritional needs. Seafood, dairy products, and leafy greens are good sources of calcium; sunshine helps the body produce vitamin D.

Adults and seniors must engage in weight-bearing exercises and resistance training to preserve their bone density and strength. These workouts help to reverse the normal decline in bone mass that occurs with age. Additionally, modifying lifestyle factors like quitting smoking and drinking excessive amounts of alcohol have a significant effect on bone health in general.

Regular bone density examinations become more crucial as people age because they allow for early detection of potential issues and timely action. Doctors may recommend calcium and vitamin D supplements if food intake is insufficient. This emphasizes how important it is to provide patients with care that is tailored to their particular health situation.

Addressing Gender-Specific Needs:

It is necessary to comprehend the aspects of osteoporosis that are unique to each gender to create dietary plans that are specifically tailored to avoid the condition. Women are more vulnerable to hormonal changes that affect bone density, especially those who have experienced menopause. Getting adequate calcium and vitamin D from food or supplements becomes essential.

Men should maintain consistent levels of testosterone since it contributes to the preservation of bone mass. Strong bones are part of a general health-promoting diet that includes lean protein, fruits, vegetables, and healthy grains.

Education about dietary requirements and gender-specific risk factors must be given top priority in preventive measures. Individualized treatment regimens ensure a comprehensive approach to osteoporosis prevention, promoting stronger and healthier bones throughout time, regardless of a person's gender. A comprehensive approach to addressing gender-specific osteoporosis preventive needs includes regular physical examinations, bone density tests, and lifestyle adjustments.

CHAPTER TWELVE

CREATING LONG-TERM OSTEOPOROSIS PREVENTION PRACTICES
Sustainability of Dietary Modifications:

Establishing enduring eating habits that will eventually prevent osteoporosis requires making decisions that can be kept up for a long period. Rather than just sticking to short fixes, it's crucial to lead a nutrient-dense lifestyle that permeates daily activities. One of the key elements is a diet that is well-balanced and full of nutrients, such as calcium and vitamin D, which are vital for bone health. Sustainability and the viability of the chosen diet are closely linked. This could involve developing delectable recipes that incorporate nutrients that fortify bones and ensuring that the food regimen aligns with personal tastes and cultural norms.

A sustainable osteoporosis prevention diet also considers how feasible it is to obtain essential nutrients from a variety of sources. Adding additional diversity to your diet not only enhances its overall nutritional profile but also adds flexibility and enjoyment. Being inclusive reduces the possibility that people will give up on their dietary adjustments out of dissatisfaction or boredom, which eliminates ennui and encourages a sustainable approach.

Moreover, the maintenance of dietary adjustments for the prevention of osteoporosis depends on the development of lifestyle-fitting habits. To enable a more seamless transition, this may mean making changes gradually. Setting realistic goals and understanding that change is a process rather than an end product will help to promote sustainability. By incorporating these dietary changes into everyday life—such as choosing healthy snacks and including elements that support bone health in regular meals—it is ensured that the preventative strategy is a long-term commitment to overall bone health rather than a temporary cure.

Monitoring And Adjusting Your Osteoporosis Prevention Plan:

An effective osteoporosis prevention plan must be dynamic and frequently evaluated and modified. Regular evaluations of nutritional intake, dietary habits, and overall bone health are essential to this process. To ensure that nutritional needs are met regularly, food journals tracking calcium and vitamin D intake may be necessary as part of the monitoring process. Self-aware people are better able to spot patterns and areas that might need to be changed.

Bone density tests and regular medical checks are necessary to monitor bone health. These assessments provide useful information on the effectiveness of the preventative plan and assist in the early detection of any potential issues. It could be necessary to adjust the preventative plan to include more physical exercise, adjust the diet, or add supplements. Consulting with medical professionals, such as doctors or dietitians, ensures that any adjustments are well-researched and tailored to the individual's requirements.

The things that work for you now might not work in the future because lifestyle and health are dynamic. The effectiveness of a preventive strategy for osteoporosis might be affected by age, general health, and living circumstances. It's important to remain flexible and realize that long-term success hinges on maintaining optimal bone health.

Acknowledging Success and Preserving Motivation:

Celebrating successes of all sizes is necessary to develop long-term osteoporosis prevention strategies. When achievements are recognized and celebrated, such as maintaining a regular exercise regimen or hitting nutritional targets, positive behavior is perpetuated. This positive reinforcement strengthens the incentive needed to sustain long-term practices.

Sustaining motivation requires setting realistic and achievable goals and breaking down more difficult tasks into smaller, more manageable ones. Respecting these benchmarks for development fosters a sense of accomplishment and boosts trust in the preventative strategy.

Incorporating enjoyable activities into the osteoporosis prevention regimen, such as engaging in bone-healthy and fun physical activities, also increases motivation.

It is crucial to have social support to stay motivated. Sharing successes with loved ones or support networks promotes a feeling of community and encouragement. Having a support system helps with accountability and motivation throughout difficult times. Maintaining commitment and attention is facilitated by periodically reassessing personal objectives and reminding oneself of the long-term benefits of osteoporosis prevention.

In summary, creating long-lasting habits to prevent osteoporosis involves a combination of persistent dietary changes, continual assessment and adjustment, and rewarding success to keep motivation high. This comprehensive approach not only satisfies immediate dietary needs but also establishes the foundation for long-term bone health.

CONCLUSION

Inspiration for a Better Tomorrow:

To sum up, adopting an osteoporosis-preventative diet is a lifestyle decision that, as opposed to being a band-aid solution, can have a lasting, significant effect on a person's overall health. Encouraging individuals to view this eating plan as an investment in their long-term health is essential. A diet rich in nutrients not only lowers the risk of fractures and the effects of osteoporosis but also increases general vigor, vitality, and resilience to a variety of health problems.

It is important to remind people that every wise choice they make now fortifies their future selves. For those who might find it challenging to change their diet or engage in regular exercise, this support is especially crucial. Small, long-lasting improvements over time can have a big positive impact on bone health and overall quality of life.

Ultimately, implementing a preventative diet for osteoporosis is a proactive step toward ensuring a stronger and healthier future. Following these dietary recommendations empowers individuals to take charge of their bone health and fosters a sense of personal responsibility for their well-being. Our research on diet-based osteoporosis prevention indicates that taking care of your bones now will result in a healthier, more resilient you down the road.

www.ingramcontent.com/pod-product-compliance
Lightning Source LLC
Chambersburg PA
CBHW060757260726

48660CB00002B/660